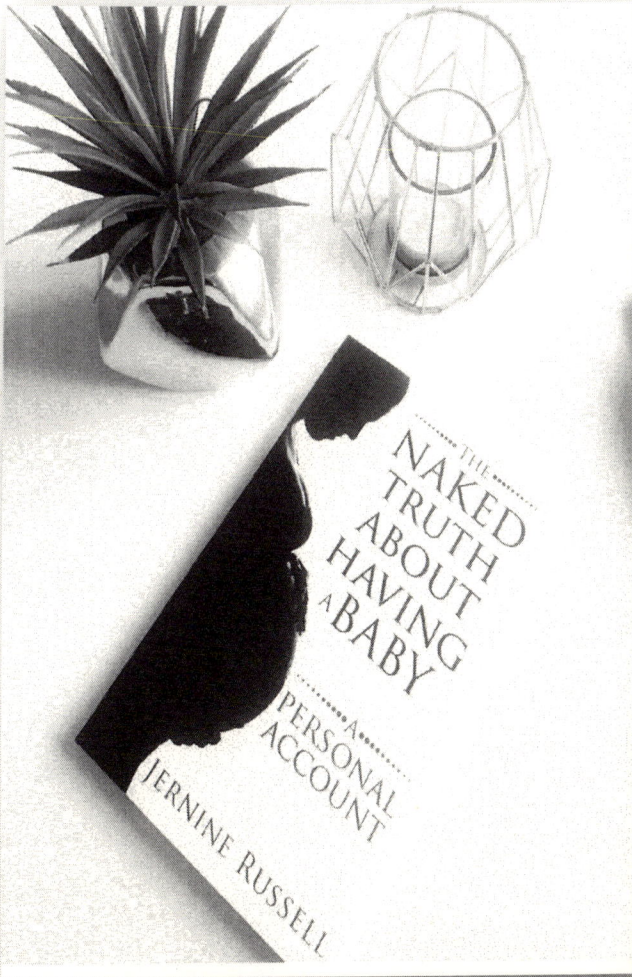

THE NAKED TRUTH ABOUT HAVING A BABY

A PERSONAL ACCOUNT

JERNINE RUSSELL

The NAKED Truth About Having A Baby

Reviews of 'The Naked Truth About Having A Baby'

"An honest and very relatable personal account, it brought back so many memories and dilemmas I faced with my first baby. It's a must read."

Founder of Prosperitys - Organisation providing practical and emotional support to expectant mums.

"I found it very relatable, particularly the chapter about the Naked Truth About Yourself. I really resonated with every word in this chapter. The Naked Truth About Childcare .... So glad that the author touched on this because I was clueless about it all. I think *The Naked Truth About Having a Baby* is informative and gives good insight to readers about the options and challenges of it all."

G.S, mother of two

"A great guide for new mums"

B.N, mother of one

"I thought it was great, in some instances I felt like I could have wrote it! It related to me so much. Nice to read something relatable."

T.H, mother of two

"A concise, yet insightful account of a woman's journey into motherhood. *The Naked Truth About Having A Baby* lays bare the glamorous and not so glamorous aspects of pregnancy and childbirth whilst giving some home truths about how life actually changes when the new baby comes home. This is a book that you can refer to every step of the way and even come back to a year down the line. I loved the realism in the author's written perspective of how things really are, from finances, to not allowing yourself to fall victim to the gadgets and gizmos, brands and old wives tales that we are all too often surrounded by once we also embark on the journey of motherhood."

Y. G, Doctor and mother of two

"I started to read and could not put it down. It is truly a lovely book and one that I really needed. I wish I had it 42 years ago!! It is written beautifully."

R.R, *Mother of two, Grandmother of six*

"Although I am not a mother, it gave me a different perspective on the actual experience of motherhood. It's an easy to swallow guide book, lots of very handy every day advice, that I would not have even thought of. I found it interesting how by reading a book you can actually have someone taking you by the hand and explaining what to do, not only what is good for the baby but also for you as a new mum. Really enjoyed it and I believe it can be such a great tool for any woman preparing to be a mum. Men – please don't pass it by, you can easily learn how to help your partner and understand what she might be going through in that life changing time, serve her by reading it and knowing a thing or two more than you already have!"

M.N

THE NAKED TRUTH ABOUT HAVING A
BABY

First published in the United Kingdom by
She Reigns Ltd, 2017

Manufactured in the United Kingdom by She
Reigns

www.she-reigns.com

Cover Design by Les Solot

Cover Image © depositphoto.com

Edited by Molah.Media

ISBN – 978-1-5272-1289-3

The NAKED Truth About
Having A Baby

Jernine Russell

Dedication

Thanks to my heavenly Father for giving me the vision to write this book.

To my husband Marlon for believing in me when I didn't believe in myself and continually encouraging me to get the book published.

To my children Reiley, Raé and Roman for your unwavering love and being the reason that I strive to be better.

To my mother for always being by my side with her love, selflessness, guidance and support in everything I do.

To my father for being the calm within the storm.

To my grandmother for introducing me to my heavenly Father.

To my siblings Bjorn and Margaret for always having my back.

To my book club ladies for reading the book, providing your constructive feedback and inspiring me to read more.

Our book club has not only enlightened and uplifted me but also made me walk towards my purpose.

To my 'ten cone' ladies, you have been a source of joy, laughter and light and have shown me so much love and understanding in the short space of time that I have known you. Thanks for believing in and supporting me.

To my friends who make me smile and love me just as I am. You know who you are.

Thanks to Esther (Pax Media) for the pictures and to my models Chanel, Victoria and baby Mireya. Thanks to Karla for helping me type the text all those years ago.

A big thanks to my mentor Carol for kicking my behind and making me see the greatness within me, and to Rhoda for editing my writing.

Thanks to Pastor Junior, Sister Sharlene and my Faith City Church family for your prayers, love and wisdom. You are a constant reminder that I can do all things through Christ our Lord.

Preface

It has been laid on my heart to write about and share my experience of becoming a mother. Before having children I would never have understood any of the emotions, life changes, stresses, joys and woes that motherhood would bring. In hindsight, I wished someone had told me the truth about what having a baby and becoming a mother really meant.

When I was in the thick of it (and I still am), I thought I was the only person going through these changes despite the fact that there are millions of other mothers in the world. Up to and during my pregnancies, all of the books I had read and all the people I had spoken to presented a sunny picture of the journey into
motherhood without actually 'keeping it real.'

With this book I want to offer just that – a real perspective on what it means to have a child. I want to give an honest and open account of one of the most wonderful, life-changing experiences you will ever have, and perhaps help you prepare for what is a lifelong journey. Maybe it may lead you to delay having a child; whichever way, I want it to contribute positively towards making the right decision for you.

By no means will this be a negative representation of motherhood, or an attempt to taint the experience of becoming a mother. It will be nothing but an honest, realistic and holistic approach to allow you to prepare for your life to change forever.

I wish you nothing but the best!

Jernine

Author Biography

Jernine is a mother of three and on a journey of re-discovering herself. She has spent the past 15 years working with disadvantaged and disenfranchised young people as a youth worker, then with both young and adult offenders as a probation officer. After a tough transition into motherhood in 2007, she felt compelled to share her thoughts and feelings with other first time mothers using one of her many skills: writing.

Fear, self-doubt and more babies meant that it took her ten years to complete this first book. Despite the arduous task of juggling motherhood, a husband and a challenging job, she persevered to get it to publication, and along the way founded the company She Reigns. She Reigns' core values are to empower, uplift and encourage others to reach their potential and realise their dreams.

The NAKED Truth About Pregnancy

The NAKED Truth About Labour

The NAKED Truth About Baby Essentials

The NAKED Truth About Bringing Baby
Home

The NAKED Truth About Sleep

The NAKED Truth About Breastfeeding

The NAKED Truth About Eating, Diet And
Weight Gain

The NAKED Truth About You

The NAKED Truth About Going Back To
Work

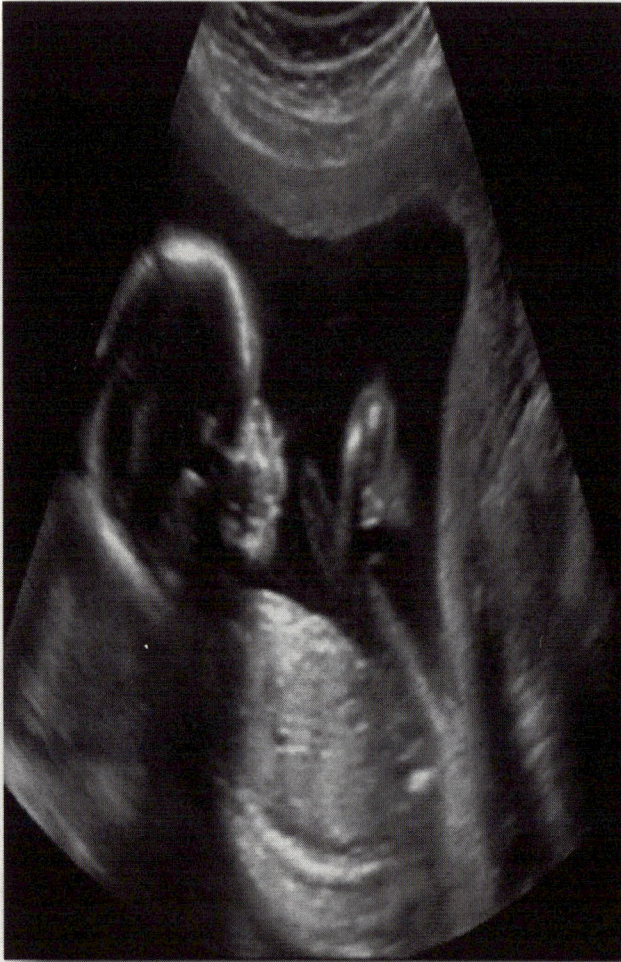

The NAKED Truth About Pregnancy

The naked truth about pregnancy is that it is the miraculous start of an incredible journey.

When I discovered that I was to become a mother for the first time, I cried. There was no real reason why I did. I can only put it down to shock...and fear. Shock because I really had no idea that I was pregnant and fear because I was venturing into the unknown.

I recalled feeling really lethargic and lacking motivation to get up and do the things I usually did. I was always full of energy and on the go. At the time I remember describing how I felt to a few friends with children; the first thing they advised me to do was a pregnancy test. In denial, I paid a visit to my doctor and told him my symptoms and he too told me the same. So up to the point of actually doing the test, I really did not expect it to be positive. I kept reading the test kit instructions over and over to be sure I had done and interpreted it correctly. Yes, two blue lines did really mean I was pregnant! Then the questions started tumbling around in my head:

Was I ready? What would my family say? How would my partner react?

The next few weeks were primarily spent trying to answer the first question as I came to the realisation that there was a tiny little life growing inside me. When I think about the intricacies of the process of conception, I am convinced that having a baby can only be a gift from God. How can it not be, especially as it can land on you just like that, without you even putting a thought to it? My partner and I had definitely not been planning to have a baby, and as a result, I had to trawl the internet to try and work out when the baby was due so that I could work out at what stage of development he or she was.

It felt like an eternity until the first scan was done, especially as I wanted to wait for the results before I told anyone outside my immediate family. I was filled with excitement, anxiety and fear. When I saw the image on the screen it confirmed what up to then had felt like a figment of my imagination. Now it was real. I kept the scan printout inside my diary and a picture I'd taken of the printout as a screen saver. I was just so in awe of *my* baby.

Needless to say, pregnancy comes with a lot of changes, not least of all physical ones. The thing to do is to embrace these changes and take care of your body reminding yourself that you are 'cooking' a beautiful baby inside. It's not easy to start with. Initially for me my changing body meant that I looked like the one who had eaten 'all the pies.' I was no longer the slim, toned and flat-stomached woman I had worked hard to become. Now I had a pot belly which made my clothes feel tight and uncomfortable. That first trimester of pregnancy was my least favourite. The ever so slight tummy bulge meant I didn't yet look pregnant, so people weren't sure what to ask – was she pregnant or was she just putting on weight?

My saving grace was Primark because I could keep up with the latest fashion trends by buying bigger sizes to accommodate my ever changing body. My breasts doubled in size in the first few months and I had to purchase the ugly maternity (non-wired) bras which everyone advised. Since my first pregnancy, most of the high street stores now have maternity departments so keeping on trend with a bump is much easier. I would suggest that you only buy the bare minimum when it comes to maternity clothes; you will really only wear them for a few months. Invest in a few pairs of leggings as these remain comfortable even as your waistline expands. Another good buy is a pair of maternity jeans that allow you to adjust the waist to accommodate your growing bump.

As part of embracing the physical changes, I highly recommend that you document and record as much of your pregnancy as possible. The nine months may sometimes feel like nine years, but trust me when I say the time passes by quickly. Write a diary and take lots of pictures. You may not feel very photogenic at times but the pictures can create a beautiful story book for your child to

'see themselves' growing in mummy's tummy. Creating a diary for yourself is also a great way to relive wonderful memories such as the first scan image and the differing emotions you experienced. There will be times down the line when those memories will come in handy!

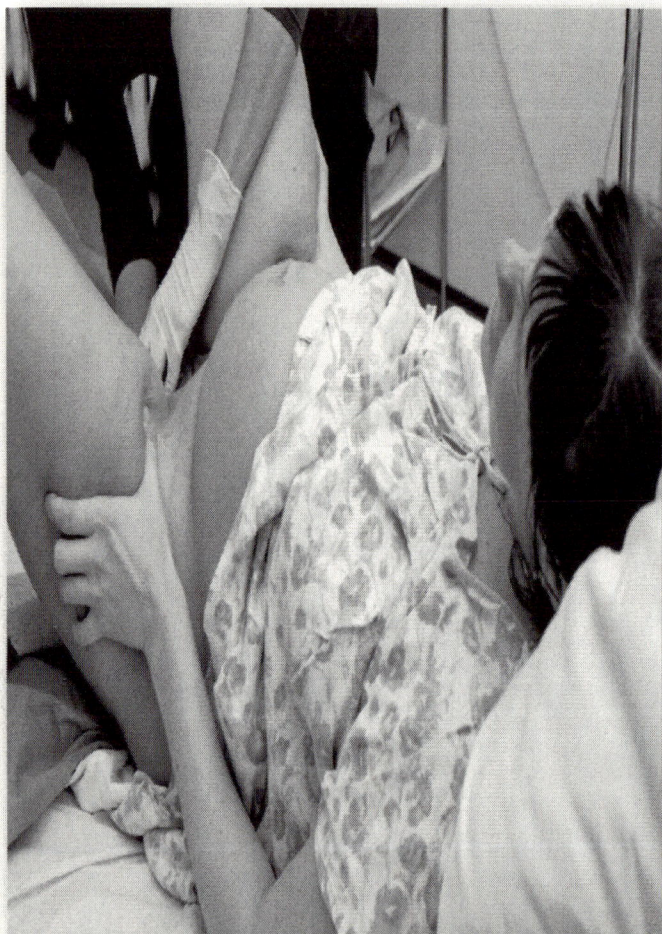

The NAKED Truth About Labour

The naked truth about labour is all in the name:
labour [ley-ber] -noun, verb, adjective - physical
toil; to work hard; of or relating to
workers

Like everyone else, I had heard my fair share of horror stories about labour, but more so whilst I was pregnant. Why everyone had to wait until it was too late for me to go back, I don't know. During one of my antenatal classes, I watched a video that just seemed so unrealistic. The fact that an actress played the part of a woman in labour didn't help. Granted, I didn't know what labour would be like but I was quite sure it wasn't as depicted in the video. I actually used to have severe menstrual cramps and my mother would always say that it was nothing compared to the pain of labour. She would say 'if you think that pain is bad, multiply it by 100.'

The truth is every woman's experience of labour is different, even right from the start when the waters break. For some, the waters gush out, for others it's a trickle and yet others may not even be aware that it has happened. With my second pregnancy, I had no idea that I had been in labour for most of the day. I was gallivanting around at my local shopping centre when I felt pain low down in my pelvis. I assumed that I was experiencing Braxton Hicks contractions (pre-labour pains). It was only on arriving home after collecting my eldest child that I decided to time the interval between the contractions especially as the pain was now persistent. After about 20 minutes, I realised that the baby was on its way and within 2 hours, she had arrived.

Here is another example of how each experience of labour is so different. My first lasted about fourteen hours, my second approximately two and a half hours and my third, six hours. The most painful of all was the third. Every woman I have spoken to says that they would much prefer a shorter labour. However, I found that with a longer labour the pain was more tolerable as the contractions were spaced out over a longer period. For me the six-hour labour was short and sharp - actually, it was excruciating! With this one, I had to admit that my mother was absolutely right about multiplying the intensity of my period pains by 100.

I like to think of contractions as waves much like the waves at a beach that rise, peak and subside as they roll towards the shore. This is exactly how they felt to me and each time a contraction started, I visualised a wave, took a deep breath in as the pain peaked, then a breath out as it eased. One of the things that really helped me was the fact that I had done yoga prior to my pregnancies. It wasn't just the physical benefits that were an advantage but also the breathing technique that I had learnt: taking deep breaths through the nose and exhaling through the mouth really worked a treat when 'riding the waves' of pain. Our natural response when in pain is to hold our breath but in actual fact taking deep breaths in and out makes it a little easier to bear.

Another piece of good advice I received during pregnancy was to listen closely to and follow the instructions of the midwife precisely during childbirth. It's really important to, even when it feels like the pain is unbearable and especially when the baby's head is crowning. This refers to the point at which the head is starting to emerge out of the vaginal canal. By this point you are in a rhythm of pushing with each contraction. However at baby crowning, the midwife will tell you to stop pushing and start panting as she/he will be manoeuvring the baby's shoulders and body out. Continuing to push at this point may cause your vaginal walls to tear.

Here is yet another take on labour. I remember sharing birth stories with one friend in particular following the birth of our first children. She had undergone a caesarean section but felt somewhat cheated that she was unable to give birth naturally (meaning a normal vaginal delivery), something I found so hard to comprehend considering the pain that I'd gone through. I often thought I may have preferred not to deal with all of that pushing and pain. My conclusion though is that whilst we expect to have a normal delivery, it's not always possible for a variety of very valid reasons. At the end of the day, the baby has to come out one way or another and as long labour ends with the safe delivery of a new life, then the method by which that happens is of little importance.

Now that the trauma of childbirth is over, it's time to finally say hello to this tiny, beautiful and miraculous being. I use the term trauma loosely of course as giving birth is by no means a negative or violent experience. For me though, the experience was emotionally and physically overwhelming and is etched in my memory forever. You would think that it would have been enough to put me off having any more children. However, once labour is over, it's over and all you want to do is meet that little person you've been carrying for nine months. Now this may sound an unusual thing to suggest, but at this time consider writing a letter to your newborn baby explaining how you feel now that you have finally met. Highlight the emotions and feelings attached to that first moment when you see the baby for the first time. Does she look the way you imagined she would? Talk about what hopes you have for his future and the impact he has already had on you. These are emotions that are best captured raw so just write as much as you can whilst the baby is sleeping in those first few hours. Imagine the fun and giggles you will have in sixteen years' time, when you share the letter with your teenager!

Let me just share a final tip for the post labour period. I wasn't prepared for the discomfort and particularly the bleeding after delivery. It was literally as if all the missed periods came at once. So, be ready and pack maternity pads and disposable underwear in your hospital bag. You will bleed for anywhere between two to six weeks so keep well stocked.

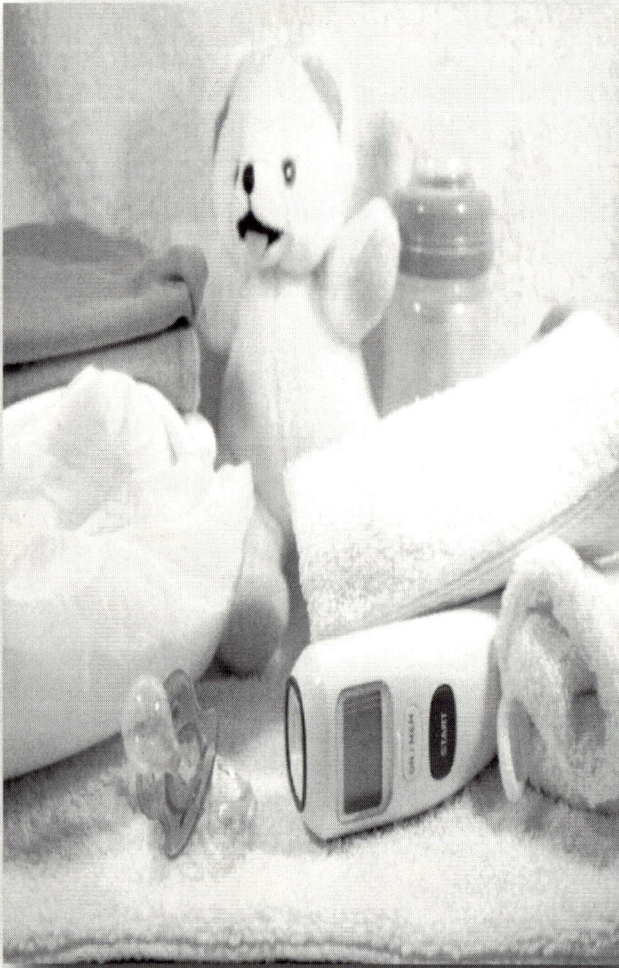

The NAKED Truth About Baby Essentials

The naked truth about baby essentials is that you have to distinguish between the things the baby needs and the things that you want.

The journey into motherhood is one of the most expensive trips that you will embark on. I would hate to think of the amount of money I have spent since becoming a mother, although, without a doubt, it's been money well spent.   Of course I had to attend a baby show during my first pregnancy. Given the opportunity, who wouldn't? It was a thrill to see these wonderful baby gadgets all under one roof and inevitably I bought a few things...well more than a few. In all honesty, I didn't use most of them when the baby finally arrived. Speaking to other parents, the general consensus is that a lot of the baby buys we make in the excitement remain unused.

Of course it's exciting to see all the amazing things in baby world and as you are entering unknown territory you want to be prepared. However, I would recommend that you make a list of the essential items with some help from other parents. In addition, borrow items from family and friends – remember they too would have some nearly new and unused items in their wardrobes! I was really fortunate as a friend lent me a lot of the essentials after the birth of my first child. One great lend was a Moses basket – all I had to do was buy a new mattress. My daughter outgrew it in two and a half months, so it was a purchase *not* well made. Finally, eBay is a great place to find items in good condition at bargain prices. I admit I was dubious about buying second-hand items for my child but after realising how quickly babies outgrow things, I was converted.

Now, to baby clothes. Despite being tempted by all the cute outfits on display, I limited myself to a starter pack of seven sleep suits and seven vests. There is no need to go overboard in the clothes department as in the initial few weeks, the baby spends most of the time in either a vest or a sleep suit. In addition, as they grow so quickly in those first few weeks, in no time, the first batch of clothes are too small. I made a point of keeping all the barely used and unworn items to give to other new mothers.

It's also now increasingly common for friends and family to throw an expectant mother a baby shower and one of my friends did just that for me. Guests are very generous with their gifts, so if you do have a shower, you may not need to buy much after that. Do wash any new clothes before the baby wears them; as baby skin is sensitive, the finish on new clothing can irritate the skin. I recall after having done my pre-birth laundry, my partner came home and was in such awe of these tiny items that he took pictures of the miniature outfits hanging on the drying rack.

Nevertheless, Mothercare and I became very well acquainted and you too will do the same with your favourite baby store. If anyone offers you gifts, I would highly recommend asking for baby store vouchers which will be useful when it comes to stockpiling on the real essentials – nappies and wipes! And, when it comes to wipes for example, it's not necessary to buy the big brands at all. I found the store brands were not only cheaper but also more absorbent. The disparity in price can be huge for not much gain in quality.

Finally, let's talk about the big ticket items – pushchairs, cots and car seats. A pushchair is one of the biggest, most exciting and crucial purchases. It's like buying a car. You want the latest model which is reliable, safe and easy to manoeuvre. Should it be a travel system that also incorporates a car seat? One of the mistakes that many new parents make is buying a huge, expensive one with all the trimmings only to end up later getting a lightweight stroller that folds up into a compact and easy-to-carry shape. Ask for recommendations from other parents. Convenience and practicality beats size and style, hands down. A cot is another big purchase for baby. We followed the advice of some of our experienced parent peers and invested in a cot bed. I am pleased to say that this item has been passed on from first baby through to the third.

A car seat is a crucial purchase especially as it's a requirement for discharge from hospital. Don't do what I did because you will end up with a *lot* of car seats. They come in different shapes for different age groups, and I made the mistake of buying a seat for each of those stages – totally unnecessary. Many brands now make car seats that last from birth to three or four years; I absolutely recommend you get one of these as it is the most cost-effective and practical option. It doesn't have to be brand new either. I bought a second hand car seat from eBay for £40 when it retails at £150. Remember that eventually you too can sell items to someone who may need them, everyone's a winner!

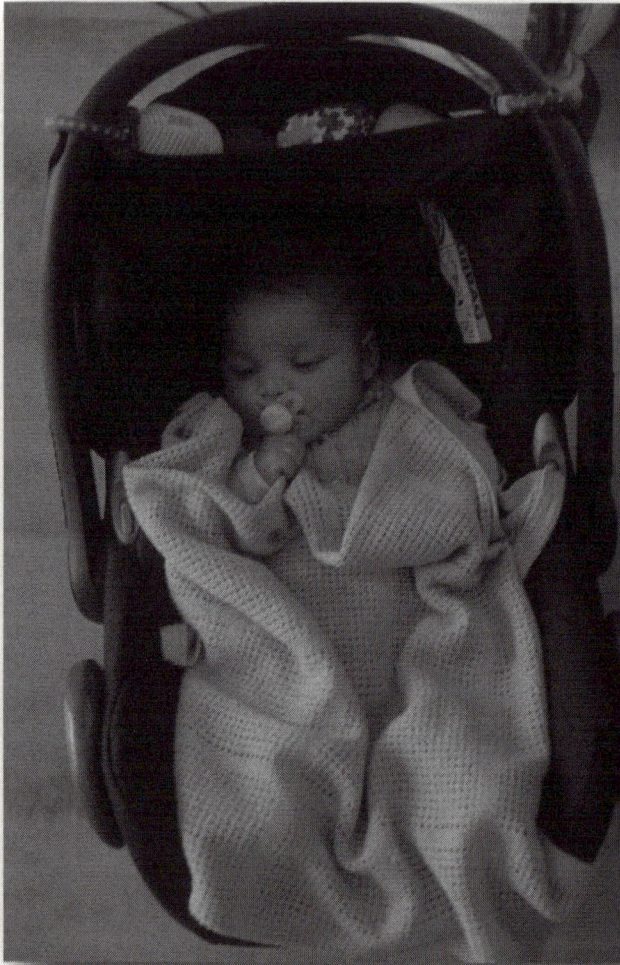

The NAKED Truth About Bringing Baby Home

The naked truth about bringing baby home is that this is where the rollercoaster ride really begins.

I can never forget bringing my eldest child home for the first time. Even though it's now almost ten years ago, I clearly recall the moment I realised that I was now responsible for another person. This tiny little thing was dependent on me. I had never felt such a weight on my shoulders. Buying a home, living on my own, paying bills - all of that paled in comparison to being responsible for the well-being of a human life.

This feeling was first and foremost compounded by the fact that the midwives were no longer there to ask questions. Even though some friends and family came to meet the new addition to the family on that first evening at home, as soon as they left I felt so vulnerable. I was way out of my comfort zone. In fact, I was in an unknown zone altogether. I felt totally out of control. Questions tumbled around in my head...again:

What if something happened to her? What if she choked? What if she stopped breathing?
Was she eating enough?

I questioned myself so much. My advice during this time would be to try and relax and tackle each new change as it comes. Don't anticipate things that may not even happen.
Just embrace it all as resistance is futile!

To be honest though, in those first few days I was an emotional wreck. One minute I'd be fine and the next I would be crying uncontrollably. No one had really warned me about the 'baby blues.' Perhaps it's difficult to explain and impossible to appreciate what it means if you've never experienced it. Whichever way, I wasn't ready. The only way to describe it was that it felt the way you would in the days leading up to a period, when the smallest thing can trigger a flood of tears. The early morning feeding didn't help either. At 3am, it seemed as if I was the only person in the whole world who was awake – a very lonely feeling.

I can't stress enough how important it is to speak to others who are going through or have already been through this phase, if only to know that you are not alone. This is where going to baby groups is so helpful. It was this feeling of being the only one going through these changes that prompted me to write this book. Communicating your feelings to those close to you can bring clarity to a situation that you are often too tired to see. A friend shared some really comforting words with me during this difficult time that I'll never forget - 'everyday gets a little bit easier' - and she was so right. In hindsight, I realised that I was just adjusting to my new role. As with all other life changes we experience, the disruption only lasts for a finite time, and during the change we have to allow ourselves time adapt.

Nevertheless, after the birth of my first child I found it almost impossible to relax. The unpredictably of the early weeks was difficult to adjust to – not knowing when she'd wake up or need a feed. I'll never forget the first time I had to go for a shower as a new mummy and not quite knowing what to do.
More questions.

Should I take her with me? What if she cries and I can't hear her?

In the end I took her into the bathroom in her car seat. In fact, during those early days, she went everywhere with me including the toilet and kitchen; basically she never left my sight. I even sat with her in the backseat of the car to keep an eye on her. We nicknamed her 'my little handbag.' Fortunately, by the time I'd had my third child, these anxieties were all gone and I could comfortably lock myself in the bathroom to escape the cries when I needed to.

Here are two other useful tips for those early days. First, invest in some anti-bacterial gel and soap so that visitors can clean their hands before handling the baby. A few years earlier, when visiting a friend after the birth of his son, I asked to hold the baby. His girlfriend abruptly asked if I had washed my hands. I felt so insulted. It was only after I became a mother myself that I understood the importance of cleanliness around newborns. They are susceptible to infections whilst their immune system is building up.

Second, get out as soon as you can. I spent the first two weeks indoors on the advice of primarily the older generation in my circle. Looking back, this didn't help my baby blues and made me anxious about going out. When I eventually summoned up the courage to go for a walk when my daughter was two weeks old, it was an overwhelming and quite frankly, a scary experience. The sound of a dog's bark and a person's cough or sneeze was amplified and I felt this powerful urge to protect my baby. I ended up rushing back home in tears, craving the sense of security of my four walls. Eventually I did feel more confident to go out with her and I noticed that when I did, she would sleep for hours afterwards and I would feel refreshed. And in those early days, when baby sleeps, mummy can relax and again, everyone's a winner! So as soon as you feel ready, go for a walk; no matter how short, just go for it.

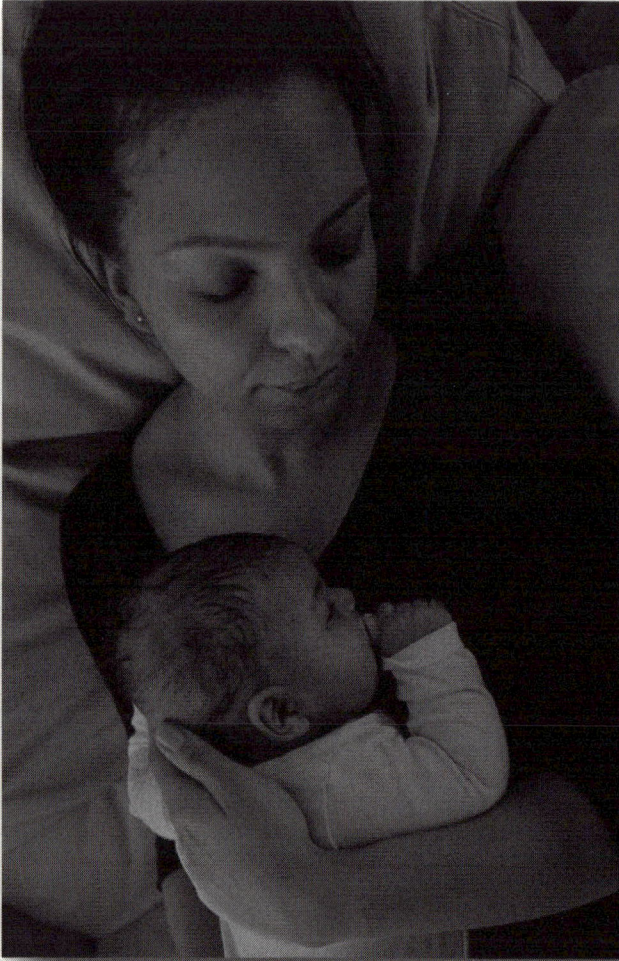

The NAKED Truth About Sleep

The naked truth about sleep is that after you have a baby you may never EVER sleep as you did before.

Sleep deprivation is, by far, one of the worst aspects of becoming a parent. It makes you snappy and irritable and yearning for uninterrupted sleep. Of course, everyone tells you to sleep when the baby is sleeping, but in reality it's not that easy to do. First time round, I would take the opportunity to tidy and catch up on chores. Second time round, I took heed and would actually lie down to breastfeed and have a nap with the baby. I'd feel so much better afterwards and was overall more relaxed. I guess I didn't feel that I had anything to prove.

In actual fact, sleep is disturbed even before the baby's arrival because during those latter months of pregnancy, your ever growing bump means you can't find a comfortable position to settle in. In addition, I developed a cramp whenever I lay in one position for too long. Perversely, it's as if the body is preparing you for what's to come.

My sleep quality and pattern changed the very first night after my first child arrived. It was very light and I felt as if I was in a state of conscious sleep. Every little move or noise my daughter made in that tiny little cot in the hospital would wake me up. Even though my children are older now, I still sleep with one ear to the ground in case they wake up. What amazes me to this day is that I can hear them even when I think I'm in a deep sleep, get up to tend to them whilst my partner remains still beside me, totally oblivious to it all (or at least that is what he wants me to believe).

To help everyone get good quality sleep, my first word of advice which you can take or leave, is to not let the baby sleep with you. There are so many reasons why it's not a good idea, the first and most important being that it can be dangerous. In addition, you'll be setting a precedent that will be very difficult to change. It's also important that the baby sleeps in their own room (if space permits). In my opinion, around nine months old is a good time to start. A new-born's sleep pattern is erratic and this is one of the things that can help them get into a routine, but you have to stick with it to make it work.

It really does take time to establish the sleep routine. In the initial stages, my first daughter would sleep all day and then wake up several times throughout the night. Other nights she would sleep for four to five hours straight and I would get my hopes up that this would be the start of her sleeping through the night. Oh, how wrong I was! I was very fortunate though in that from the age of six weeks she did sleep through the night. I really do think that this was largely down to my mother's advice to establish a routine. For us, that involved a bath consistently around 8-8:30pm, dressing up in pyjamas followed by a feed, then soon after, straight to bed. However, each baby is different. My son, who is now three years old, still wakes up during the night. This can be draining because even though he goes back to sleep, my sleep is interrupted and it can sometimes take a long time for me to drift off again.

I also faced a dilemma that most first time mothers have to face: whether to place the baby on their tummy, back or side to sleep. My mother told me that 'in her day' they were advised by doctors and midwives to lay babies on their tummies; however my midwife advised me that the current research at the time supported putting a baby to sleep on its back. I was conflicted because I respected my mother's advice but wanted to follow medical guidance as well. In the end I compromised and put my daughter to sleep first on her tummy during one of her daytime naps allowing me to observe her sleep which she did for six straight hours! As she appeared to be safe, I continued to put her to sleep in this position. To this day she sleeps on her tummy. I'm inclined to think that she learnt to hold her head up quickly and crawl at an early age as she was so accustomed to lying prone. However, with these things, always be guided by medical advice, but don't necessarily dismiss your own opinions.

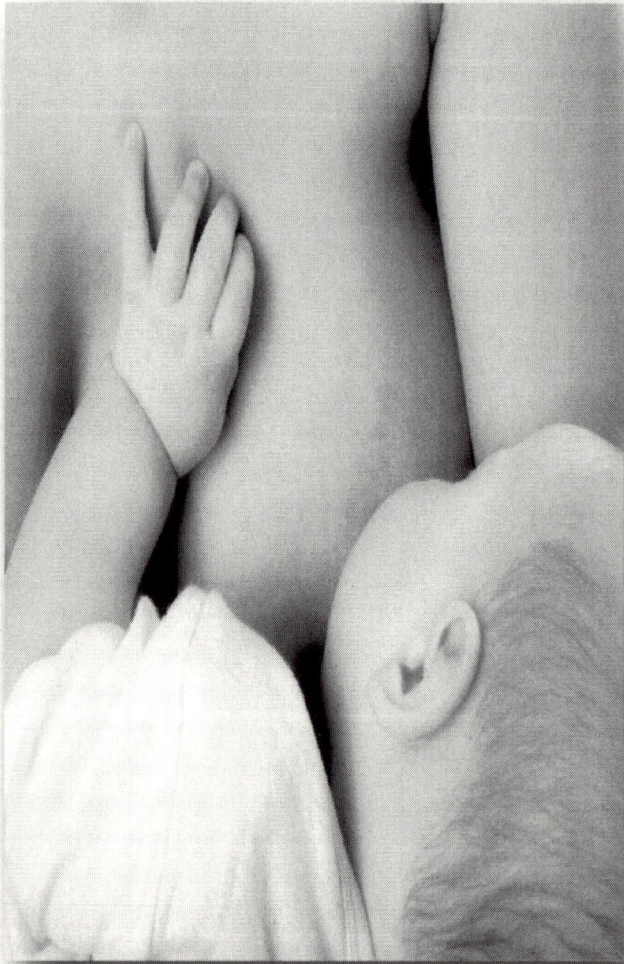

The NAKED Truth About Breastfeeding

The naked truth about breastfeeding is that it sometimes requires hard work and perseverance.

Breastfeeding. Some babies take to it while others don't. Some women find it difficult while for others it comes quite naturally. 'Breast is best' is a saying that is all too familiar. This was certainly the advice I was given by the doctors and midwives as well as friends and acquaintances with children. I must say though that one friend almost put me off as she was still breastfeeding her daughter right up to the point of her starting school!

One of the benefits of breast milk is that it's readily available, free and convenient. Feeding at night is easy as you don't have to get up and prepare a bottle. I just picked the baby out of the Moses basket, fed and winded her whilst I lay in bed, then put her back to sleep. Another benefit of breastfeeding is weight loss. I lost the 'baby weight' after my first child quickly; apparently breastfeeding burns a lot of calories.

I breastfed all of my children but the experience was different each time. Breastfeeding for the first time was a daunting, exhausting and tedious task. In the early post-natal period, the breasts produce what is called colostrum, or first milk, which contains anti-bodies to protect the new-born against disease. It takes a few days for real milk to express but once it does believe me when I tell you that you feel it. My breasts hurt tremendously every time my daughter latched on. Looking back, this was perhaps partly due to her not being positioned properly on my breasts leading to sore nipples.

Throughout my pregnancies the midwives advised me that in order to make breastfeeding easier to initiate, I should ensure that the baby is placed straight onto my skin after birth. This didn't happen with my first daughter as she was taken away for checks before being given to me. I still wonder if this may have been the reason I found it difficult to breastfeed her. There were times I would feed her for an hour on each breast after which she would scream in apparent hunger – it was as if I hadn't fed her at all. On top of that I was the only person who could feed her. My partner tried to ease the pressure and suggested that I express milk allowing him to feed our daughter. That would frustrate me no end, as I could just about feed her let alone express.

There was a crucial point in that first experience of breastfeeding where my daughter was very unsettled, appeared to be constantly hungry and cried endlessly despite me breastfeeding her on demand. Strangely enough, it was my brother who helped the most during that time. He suggested that I was having difficulty producing milk because I wasn't eating or drinking enough. He was right, because I was actually finding it difficult to make time to eat. I hadn't been aware of the fact that inadequate food intake and in particular liquid could impact on my ability to breastfeed. Sure enough, when I started eating regularly and drinking plenty of water I noticed a marked difference in the quality of our breastfeeding routine.

In the end I did have to combine breast- with bottle-feeding. My first shopping trip for formula was a revelation. There was an array of different brands all claiming to be the closest thing to breast milk and packed with nutrients and vitamins. I had no idea where to start so I phoned a friend. I'd picked up one particular brand, though I wasn't sure why, and during our conversation she told me that she had used that same one. That at least reassured me that I'd made the right choice!

As a matter of fact, I was quite emotional during our phone conversation. Even though I had reconciled with the fact that bottle feeding was necessary, I still felt a failure for not being able to breastfeed exclusively. She of course countered my claim explaining that more parents than we

56

think have to bottle-feed their babies, that at least I had tried hard, but that what was ultimately best for the baby was to be well fed and content. I still waited another week after that conversation before I gave her the first bottle. Lo and behold, I immediately noticed a change in my daughter – she was indeed content. The tension eased as I was no longer the only one who could feed her. I went on to alternate breast with bottle for 2 months, all the time seeking advice from a midwife on how I could improve on breastfeeding. She gave such good advice that I regretted not having sought help earlier. I also attended a weekly breastfeeding group and was encouraged by the stories that the other mothers shared with me.

Breastfeeding my second and third child was a completely different experience. I thoroughly enjoyed it, felt relaxed and so bonded very well with them during feeding. I often wonder if part of what made it easier was having that immediate skin-to-skin contact after birth. Undoubtedly the fact that I felt more confident and secure in my skills as a mother also helped. As a result I was able to pass on the same advice about eating well, drinking plenty of water and mix feeding that I'd received to a family friend who was experiencing the same challenges with her baby boy that I'd had with my first daughter.

There were two incidents during the breastfeeding part of the journey that were a major cause of concern for me. In hindsight I wish someone had warned me. When I took my first baby for a weigh-in one week or so after she was born, the midwife told me that she had lost weight. I was immediately concerned that I might have been doing something wrong. But the midwife explained that it was quite common for babies and especially those that are breast-fed to lose weight in the initial weeks. This is because they lose fluid in those first few days when they are first exposed to the outside world. As their stomachs are tiny, they cannot take in enough milk to make up for the fluid loss, but they soon adjust.

The second 'emergency' arose after my daughter hadn't passed a poo for 3 days. I hadn't been particularly worried until I went to visit an older family member, who put the 'frighteners' in me telling me to take her to the doctors straight away - which I duly did. The first thing the doctor asked was, 'Is this your first baby?' I found myself hearing that phrase often whenever I attended a doctor's appointment. It was only after consulting a breastfeeding midwife that I got an explanation for 'poo-gate,' it was quite normal for a breastfed baby to go anything up to seven days without passing a poo.

So my final word of advice is that should you have difficulties with feeding, get help early. Midwives run breastfeeding clinics in many health centres so take advantage of these. It doesn't matter if you think your concerns are minor. The fact is this is new territory for you and there is a lot to learn. Breastfeeding is just another of those things on the list to get to grips with.

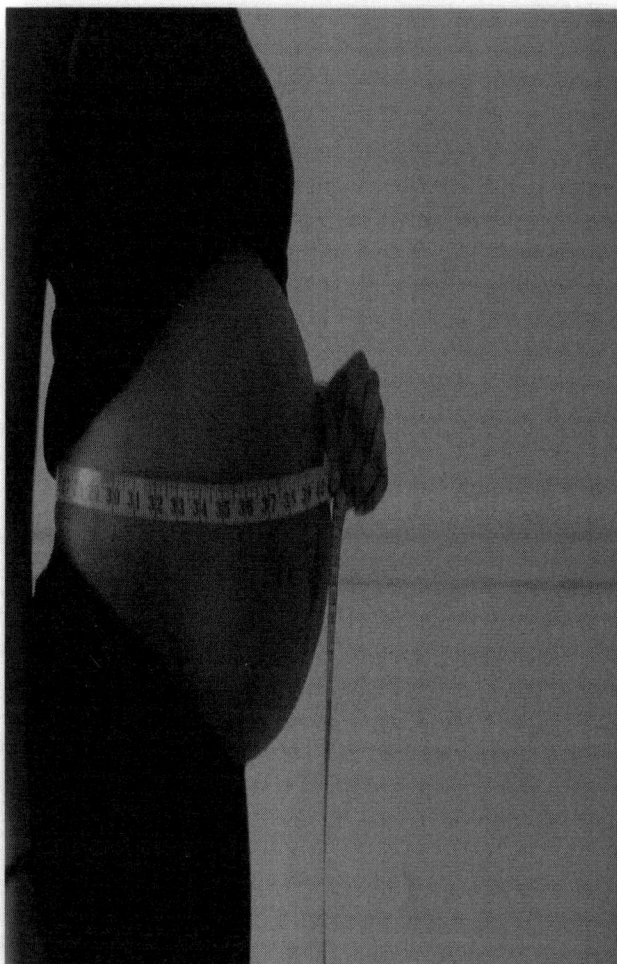

The NAKED Truth About Eating, Diet And Weight Gain

The naked truth about weight during pregnancy is that though it goes up, it can always come down.

Gaining weight is inevitable during pregnancy. Your body is housing a new life that is growing rapidly. As with all the other changes I can only recommend that you embrace your body's transformation. Believe me when I say that you won't see your genital area or toes for a while!

There are lots of 'dos and don'ts' about what you should eat. As I've said before, follow medical guidance but don't disregard your own opinions. The core advice on diet in pregnancy is to actually eat healthily, but certainly not for two. Then of course there are the cravings! During my first pregnancy, I had a particular taste for cheese (I still wonder if that is why my daughter dislikes cheese so much). With my second pregnancy, I really craved junk food although I did control how much of it I ate. With my third pregnancy I ached for spicy food, though I could only eat it once the nausea had subsided.

Speaking of nausea, morning sickness is a hot topic of discussion for expectant mothers. It's a misnomer because according to most of the women I know, it more often than not lasts way past the morning. Some experience it throughout the whole day. Others found they struggled to eat, whilst for others, food actually helped. However, for most it really does subside around the three month mark. Unfortunately for a minority, it lasts for most of the pregnancy. I felt as if I was on a boat for three months and my relief came from satsumas. I always had to have a stash in my handbag!

Let's talk about weight loss. First of all, the one thing to avoid at all costs is to be influenced by the images of celebrities who revert to a size 0 immediately after having a baby. Remember, they don't live in the real world because they usually have a personal trainer, chefs preparing their meals and nannies caring for their new-borns. They have all the time in the world to 'kill' themselves to get back into shape...as well as sleep! Just don't give in to the pressure to lose weight quickly.

The reality of losing weight after having a baby is that again, the experience is different for everyone. After my first pregnancy, I lost weight in no time perhaps because I hadn't gained much more than the weight of the baby. Within two weeks I was back into my pre-pregnancy jeans without exercise. With my second pregnancy, the weight was harder to shift so after six to seven weeks, I had to start exercising.

The truth is that you have to work to get to a place where you are happy with your physical appearance after having a baby. If you're not, do something about it. I didn't like my tummy so I did more sit ups than I used to. It may not be so easy to lose that belly after having a caesarean section though but it's not impossible. The truth is losing the baby weight is not just for celebrities, it's just that for us normal folk it takes a little bit more time and a lot of patience.

My advice would be to start your weight loss programme after you have been given the all clear from your GP at your six week check, and especially if you had a caesarean section. Don't forget that is a major operation. Eating and exercising should be done in moderation. Follow a balanced diet and remember that starving yourself will not help. Drink lots of water. When it comes to exercise, you can start by taking short walks with the baby, increasing the intensity and frequency slowly. I had never walked so much until I had children. It's also really helpful to find an activity that you enjoy and that fits into your routine. After my second pregnancy, I took part in an exercise class once a week and my 'fun' activity was trampolining. I still do a weekly circuit class and swim to help maintain a healthy weight. One bonus that comes with exercise is that you get 'me' time, something that's hard to come by as a mother!

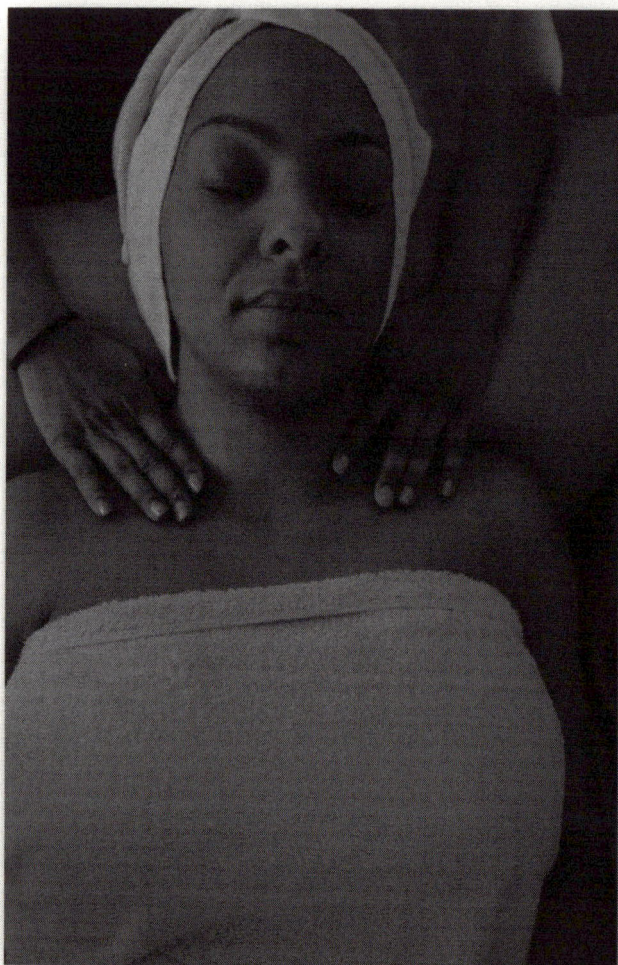

The NAKED Truth About You

The naked truth about you is that after having a baby, you will neither be physically nor mentally the same again.

The physical changes of pregnancy are of course obvious and need no explanation, although I do marvel at the way a woman's abdomen and breasts are able to stretch and bounce back to size, (though not back to the same shape). My breasts for example are nowhere near as perky and upright as they used to be. I have to wear a bra all the time now!

The real lasting changes though are mental, psychological and personal. Perhaps these changes are necessary as you are now fully responsible for another human life and that in itself is a whole new ball game. There are so many life lessons that come with motherhood and in the process, you learn much about yourself. Having to prioritise someone else's needs over yours leads to selflessness. I fully comprehend the meaning of sacrifice now especially as going out every weekend and blowing £100 on a pair of shoes are firmly things of the past. I have also learnt to be more patient. Being a mother has also made me more insightful and I can honestly say that I have a more holistic view on life.

As the focus is no longer on you, inevitably it is difficult to find time for yourself. I recommend making a conscious effort to make this time. One way to do this especially in the early weeks, even with all the apparent chaos, is to get out and get your hair and nails done, simply as a pick me up. If you have a good support network, and as your baby gets older, try and spend a few hours on your own just to recharge and refresh.

It actually becomes difficult to recall what life was like before you had a baby. It's almost as if you've lost a little piece of yourself. It wasn't until I went back to work that I felt like myself again because at work I had my identity. I wasn't Reiley's mum - I was Jernine! I could sit down and take my time to eat lunch rather than grabbing a quick bite in between feeding the baby and putting in a load of laundry. Remember you will be dealing with little people who have no awareness of you being anything else but their mother, whose sole purpose is to meet their every need. I still can't get over the fact that my children think that they have a right to come into the toilet even while I'm doing a poo! They follow you everywhere, so going back to work allows you space - a refreshing feeling.

Prior to having children I was generally quite fearless. However, after babies this changed. I recall a visit to the theme park Alton Towers where I queued up for 2 hours for one ride, only to chicken out at the last minute and just as the attendant was about to put the safety bar over me. I would never have done that before - I would have gone on any ride there was without a moment's hesitation. Now as a mother I tend to analyse situations more carefully as ultimately my decisions no longer affect just me.

My memory is no longer the same either, and 'baby brain' is very real. I noticed the change during pregnancy and it continued unabated after I had the children. I do wonder if it's all down to having so much more to think about and remember and organise when it comes to caring for a child. At the same time you continue to run a home, juggle life and its twists and turns, and all on a background of sleep deprivation! It's known that the hormonal changes during and after pregnancy do have an effect on cognitive function, but all that the brain has to process as a parent must also play a role!

Going through change and having to learn new skills also takes its toll on your confidence. I can testify that it took some time for me to get back to being the vibrant and bubbly character I was before my children. I was always trying new things, full of vitality and thirsty for new experiences. However, becoming a mother did come with a lot of self-doubt. For example, I have wanted to write about my experiences of motherhood since my daughter was born in December 2007. It has taken me ten years to do it. But here I am with a published book. The truth is that if you are learning a new set of skills, it takes time to master them (if you can say that you ever master being a mother, you just do the best you can). Just as it took time for you to learn enough in school and/or university to obtain your qualifications, and master the skills required for your job, so must the same happen with motherhood. Despite that initial loss of confidence as a new mother, you do gain new skills and develop different qualities, all of which make you a better person.

Becoming a mother forced me to rediscover and value time with myself. Before the children, I never fully appreciated spending time in my own company. There is nothing I love more now than being on my own sitting in the park. I really appreciate the quiet time to think and reflect. For a period after having my second child I lost my balance and control and it felt as if I loved everyone else more than I loved myself. One weekend I decided to go away. I ensured my children were in good hands so that I wouldn't worry. During that time, I had a lot of time on my own to think and make plans for my future. I did some shopping because there's nothing better than retail therapy as a pick-me-up. Just spending some time catching up on sleep and reading, two things I had missed sorely with the multiple interruptions that come with having children, went a long way to restoring that lost balance.

Despite the journey into motherhood being a bumpy one, I wouldn't change it for the world. I have grown more than I ever could, am much calmer and I don't sweat the small stuff anymore. I prioritise what's and who's important. My friendship circle is more diverse but in the main, most of my peers have children and so our priorities are matched. Friends without children understand that my children come first but know that I will make time for them. The secret to embracing the new you lies in seeking balance in everything you do.

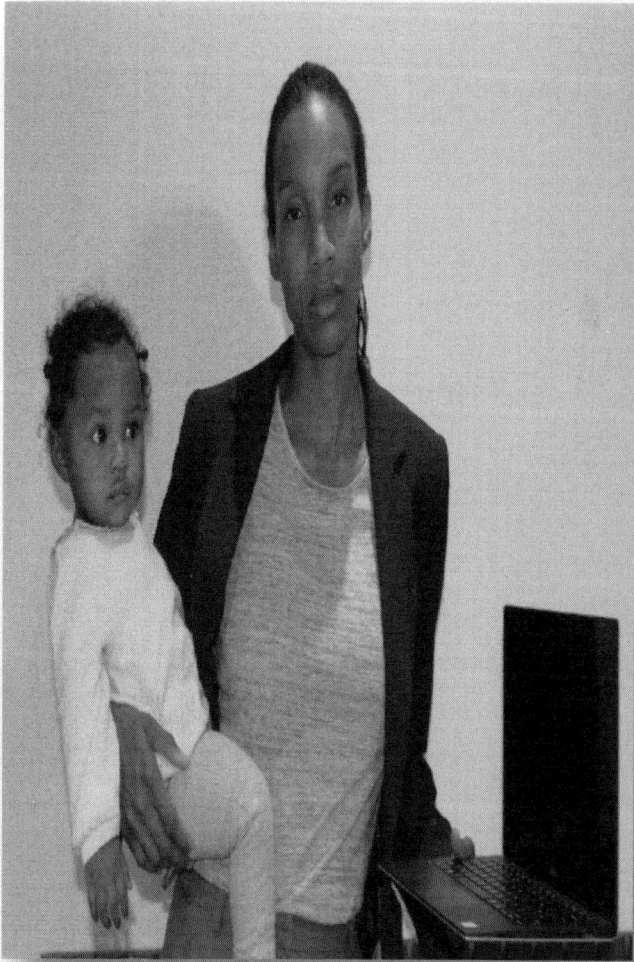

The NAKED Truth About Going Back To Work

The naked truth about going back to work? It has its pros and its cons.

I had mixed feelings about returning to work after having my children but knowing that I had bills to pay absolutely influenced my decision. If you are planning to have a child it may be an idea to start a savings scheme to ensure you are able to cover your living costs whilst you are not at work. Babies are expensive! In the early days, you will find yourself frequently meeting with friends for lunch as well as getting yourself little treats. All this needs money, and you will be surprised by how much it all adds up. Maternity pay does differ depending on where you work and how long you have been with your employer. I knew of someone who had six months full pay whilst others didn't have that option at any point for any period of time.

If you become a housewife, it's not a bad idea to do so for as long as possible. The benefits of staying home with the growing child are multiple. You experience the pleasure of watching them as they develop and meet their milestones. You also don't have to worry about anyone else caring for your child. The disadvantages are that things may be tight financially without your income and depending on your personal circumstances. You may also find it a little overwhelming to spend entire days caring for a little person.

Whether staying at home long-term or taking a fixed duration of maternity leave, do your homework and find out what you are entitled to so that you can plan and budget properly. I didn't do my homework, so one of the biggest shocks I got was the payslip I received six months into my first maternity leave. I remember phoning my workplace that very day asking to return earlier than planned as I realised I couldn't afford all of my outgoings.

Two things I enjoyed about returning to work were the stimulation that came with being around adults and being able to eat uninterrupted! The thing I least enjoyed was missing out on all the new things that my children were doing in my absence. Quality time with the children was limited to weekends - during the week it was (and still is) a constant hustle to get the kids to nursery (then school) and you to work, then leaving work on time to pick them up, get everyone home to be fed and washed before bed, ready for the cycle to start again the following day.

I now work four days per week allowing me to spend three days with my children. It still doesn't feel as if we have enough time together but I'm working hard to change that. Sometimes I do wonder what it would be like to stay at home full-time. However, I quickly rule this out as an option after a hectic day at
home with the endless cries of 'Mummy!'

The guilt that comes with being a working mother never really disappears. I remind myself though that I'm being a role model for my children by working to provide financial support and security for them to have ample opportunities down the line. It makes me smile when my girls pick up their little

handbags and proudly play 'going to work!'

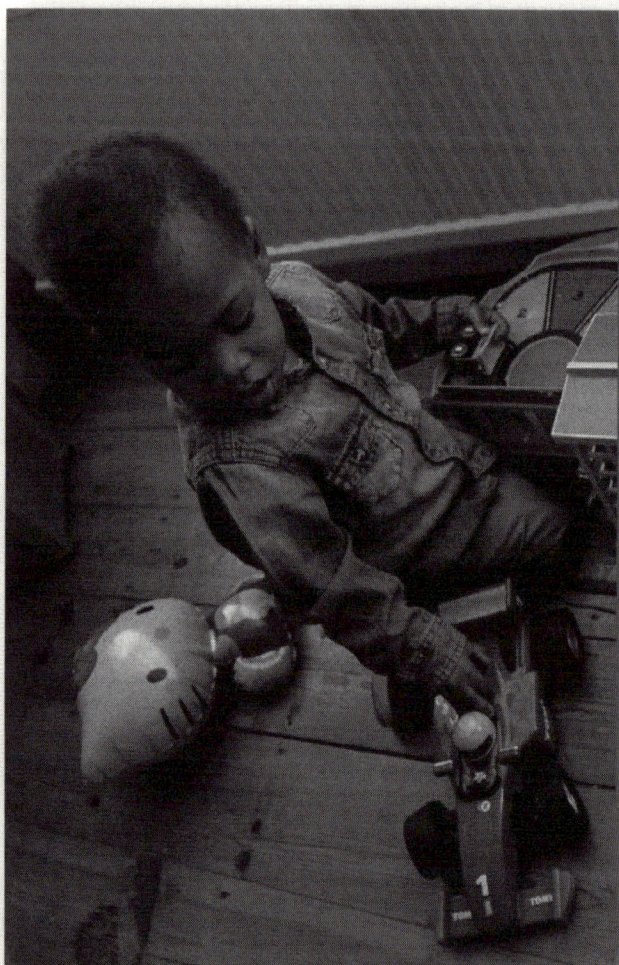

The NAKED Truth About Childcare

The naked truth about childcare is that it's expensive.

Choosing the right childcare can be a daunting experience. Whatever arrangements you eventually choose, you must feel comfortable as you are handing over the most precious thing to you into someone else's care.

When considering the different childcare options, there are a few things you need to consider - the cost, location, hours per day and length of time you need covered. It is an important decision and a big financial commitment. You will have to weigh up the cost effectiveness of working full- or part-time as the cost of full-time childcare, particularly nursery, is like paying a mortgage. You may find it more beneficial to have a nanny or an au pair caring for your child/ren in their own environment, and in return, you don't have to worry about dropping them off or picking them up at a specific time. My aunt and uncle always used au pairs which accommodated their long working hours. That arrangement also allowed them to have a social life as their support network was limited.

One thing to note is the difference between a nanny and an au pair. A nanny is a qualified childcare provider who is your employee so their salary will include tax and national insurance contributions; this can make it quite expensive. They may or may not live with you. An au pair on the other hand will not necessarily have childcare qualifications though some may. They would usually be a young person from overseas who comes to live with you for a different cultural experience in exchange for helping you with the childcare. They live in your home and you provide them with pocket money of around £80-£120 per week, depending on the number of children you have and the household duties you need help with. Another key difference is that au pairs cannot look after babies and toddlers whilst nannies can care for children of all ages. Someone I know had the best of both worlds as a relative actually lived with her family in their home caring for their children and doing the housework. This is not so easy to do these days as the immigration rules are more limiting than they used to be.

With my daughters the best choice for us was my extended family. This meant I could return to work early, especially after I discovered that shortfall between maternity pay and my bills! My god-mother and my 'extra mum' (as I affectionately call her) each cared for my daughters twice a week. After I had my third child, my mother and my mother-in-law also stepped in. These women have done an exceptional job in helping to raise the children in my absence and probably do a better job than I do at looking after them...or should I say spoiling them. I feel very fortunate for the love and support they have given my children and I, as well as the peace of mind I had knowing they were safe whilst I was at work.

With the arrival of my second daughter, I did have to make alternative childcare arrangements for the first so that she was settled into a routine before her sister arrived. I visited quite a few nurseries before I found one that I liked. There were so many to choose from. It's good to get a list of those that are accessible from where you live or alternatively where you work. Go and visit them to get a feel for the environment. Speak to other parents whose children attend the nurseries that you shortlist. Many popular nurseries now have lengthy waiting lists, so I suggest adding your child's name as early as possible. My final choice was primarily based on the attitude of the staff and their interaction with the children. Other factors that came into play were the location, the opening times, the cleanliness and the fees. However, I still had to rope in the grandmothers to collect them when I had an engagement after work or if I was running late.

It can sometimes feel as if you are the only person making important decisions for your child. However, when making these big choices, getting advice from those who have already walked the walk is extremely helpful. This is absolutely true when considering childcare and every other parent, even stay at-home mothers, have had to weigh up their options and make a choice. Personal recommendations are invaluable, especially if coming from those in your circle of friends and acquaintances as you are likely to want the same things. I was certainly able to do just that when a colleague of mine asked me what he should ask and look for at nursery visits. Fortunately for him, I was in a good position to share my experiences. And if you don't know many other parents there are multiple parenting websites with discussion forums where you can also seek advice.

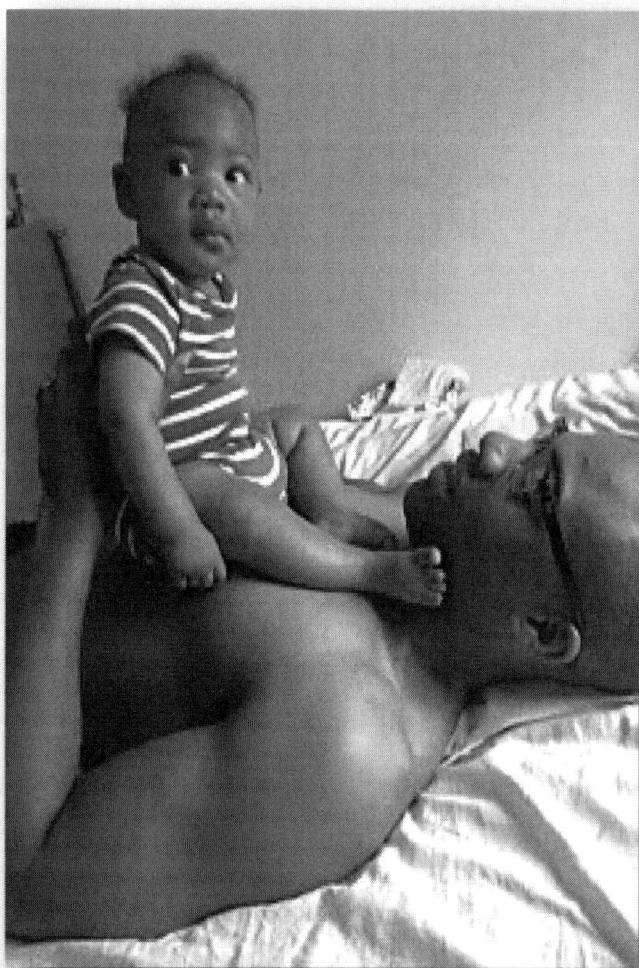

The NAKED Truth About Your Relationship

The naked truth about your partner is that he goes through changes too but in a different way. When it comes to relationships, having a baby can either make you or break you.

Having a baby really tests a relationship. So if you are already experiencing problems, please don't expect a baby to fix things. In fact, it may do exactly the opposite. Think about it, even on a very simplistic level, tending to any problems within a relationship requires time, commitment and focus. How can that happen when another life requires your full attention?

In my view, fathers have a completely different experience of becoming a parent. For one, they don't undergo the physical changes that come with pregnancy. They don't feel the kicks. They haven't had a baby shower thrown for them and they haven't had the first physical contact with this new life. So for them, reality only sinks in after the baby has arrived. They can feel quite helpless and useless during the initial stages, especially if you are breastfeeding. However, they can counter these feelings by doing the things they can do. I recommend that they change and bathe the baby right from the beginning. It can be daunting as the baby is so tiny, but with familiarity comes confidence. Fathers can also take the baby out after a feed, meaning mummy can get some well-deserved rest.

One word of advice I would offer that is based on my personal experience is to ensure that you communicate with your partner. I wasn't very good at communicating how difficult I found it to adjust to motherhood. I supressed my feelings and pretended that I had it all together. When I look back, I realise I wasn't being honest with myself or anyone else for that matter. Let your partner know how you're feeling and about your experiences of looking after the baby. It's important that men are able to understand that the baby does require a great deal of attention especially in the early days and only you can tell them how demanding a job it is. Give him the chance to know that you are learning to be a mother. You can then see how keeping the lines of communication open allows him to step in where he needs to.

In turn fathers can help by checking how their partners are coping and perhaps taking over some of the other household duties for a period. This goes a long way in alleviating some of the pressure that new mothers feel. Remember that just as you created the baby together, you must also care for the baby together.

When talking about relationships, we have to talk about sex. For obvious reasons, sex is the last thing that most new mothers think about. The body has gone through a lot during delivery and needs time to heal and rest. The medical recommendation is that we wait for at least six weeks following childbirth before engaging in sexual intercourse; this may be longer in the event of a caesarean section. It is a challenge for men to abstain from sex for such a long time but this is where men have to put their needs aside. However, couples can still be affectionate and loving and meet their sexual needs without engaging in penetrative sex. This is when patience is a real virtue.

Whilst adjusting to the new addition in the family as well as the new schedule that comes with that, please don't forget to make time for each other. It's really easy to put all your focus on the baby but remember your relationship is the means by which this child came to being and the foundation on which that child will grow. It's important to keep that foundation sturdy enough to support all that is to come in the future. Try and have a date night regularly. You can go to a favourite restaurant or after baby's bedtime have a romantic dinner at home. It's important for men to make their partners feel special and cared for because motherhood can make women lose sight of who they are in a brand new territory. Caring for a baby, sometimes with other children too, is very demanding and leaves little time to care for you. So simple gestures such as a foot massage or running a bath for her really go a long way to making her feel valued.

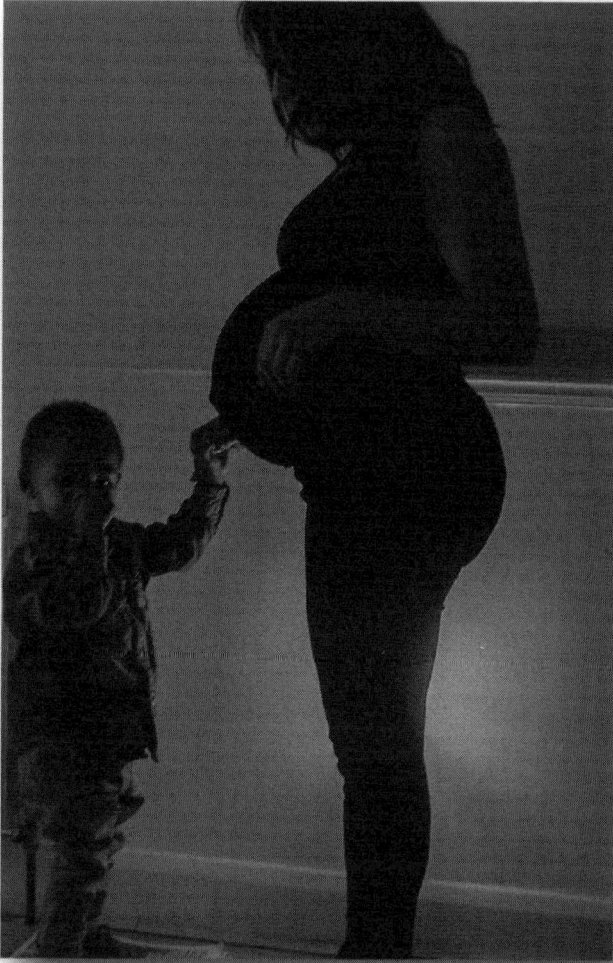

The NAKED Truth About Having Another Baby

The naked truth about having another baby is that there is never a right time to do it.

When I found out that I was expecting my second child a few days after my daughter's first birthday, I asked, 'Oh God, why?' I could barely cope with one child let alone two. When baby number two arrived, baby number one was only 20 months old. I can honestly say that caring for the both of them was one of the most difficult things that I've ever done. I found it so overwhelming and felt that I would never get through it. But of course through the grace of God that had given me a wonderful support network I did get through it. The crucial changes on my part were accepting that I couldn't do everything on my own and just asking for help.

It's only now, almost ten years later, that I'm able to look back on that period with some clarity. The conflicting demands were the biggest challenge. Baby two was being breastfed whilst baby one was being potty trained and wanting me to play with her all the time. I only managed to breastfeed baby two for four months because baby one was so jealous that she would pull my breast out of her sister's mouth! Although she would kiss and cuddle her baby sister, when our backs were turned she would bite and pinch her meaning I couldn't leave the baby out of my sight. Nevertheless, I still think I did the best thing for us by having them one after the other because they get along so well now. No one can convince me to do it all over again though!

There are some steps you can take to ease the transition from only child to big sister or brother. Involve your older child/ren with the baby from the beginning. There are some wonderful children's stories about becoming a big sister or brother which can be read throughout the pregnancy to prepare them for their new sibling. Once the baby is born, buy the older child a present from the baby and make a fuss of them too. Once at home and able, the older child can assist with nappy changes, feeds and cuddles.

Try and spend some quality, one-on-one time with the older child when the baby is sleeping. When the new baby is old enough to be left with someone else, take the older child out to their favourite place or let them stay up and watch a movie with you. All children usually want in this situation is to spend time, alone, with you.

Since the arrival of my son five years after my second child, I can also see the advantages of a bigger age gap between siblings. You end up with instant little helpers who are only too willing to help you with the baby. The older child can understand what it means to have a new baby in the home and this allows them to manage and express their emotions.

Overall, having another baby ends up being better than you might have expected. You realise how much you learnt with the first and so feel more confident and competent the second time around. Above all, it's a joy to see the different personalities interact to create a family unit.

Despite the fact that there are hundreds of books written about pregnancy and becoming a parent, very few of them tell you the raw naked truth about what it really means to have a baby. Neither does anyone tell you what the books don't. The other side of the coin is that perhaps we don't really hear the truth as the notion of a blooming pregnancy and cherubic babies that sleep peacefully is one that's so imprinted in our psyche that anything else is difficult to even consider as the reality. Or it could be that it's a life change that no one could really articulate anyway but one that has to be experienced.

I was unprepared for my first journey into motherhood and my experience inspired me to share my perspective so that you could be better prepared. For those of you already on your way and feeling a little lost, I wanted you to know that you are not alone. It's entirely up to you how you use the information and advice I have detailed throughout this book. Whatever stage you are at, I hope that my account has left you a little better informed and more equipped to handle this life changing event.

Afterword

Thank you for taking the time out to read my book. Let me add that I am not a medical professional and all the information I have shared is based on my personal experiences and opinions alone. So, why did I write this book?

Well, first of all I needed to acknowledge and share three things that I think can go a long way to ease the journey: i), motherhood can be challenging, ii), though you may feel alone during the struggles, you are not, iii), everyday gets a little bit easier. Through it all, you learn, develop and grow just as your baby does. And so with this book, I wanted to help you get through the many foggy bits and encourage you to breathe, enjoy the journey and look forward to where it may take you.

It has taken me ten years to complete this book and believe me when I say that it's an amazing feeling to be here! Why did it take so long? The honest answer is that fear and self-doubt stood in my way, because the journey is long, arduous and at times just one hard slog (and it's nowhere near done)! Under such circumstances, it's easy to lose sight of who you are and why you are where you are. I thought I had lost much but along the way I had actually acquired new skills and polished others - patience, commitment and tenacity being a few - all of which enabled me to achieve this lifelong dream. Writing this book has therefore been a way of celebrating the privilege of raising and creating memories with three beautiful children. Without them, I wouldn't have experienced and triumphed over the challenges I faced, a process that allowed me to realise my dream. On top of that, I leave a tangible legacy for those three souls.

So, I wish you well on your ride – remember no matter how bumpy it gets, embrace it fully and let it take you to heights greater than you could ever have imagined.

Letters To My Children

Dear Baby Reiley,

When I look at you, I can't believe that you were inside me. You are beautiful, with your thick black hair, almond eyes and kissy lips, just like your daddy.

Today, I thanked God for giving you to me and asked that He guide and protect us all. I know that He will bless my family and particularly my special little girl.

Thank you for changing my life. Thank you for coming into my world to teach me about myself and for inspiring and encouraging me to be the best version of myself.

Baby, I'm so glad you came into my life.

Lots of love,
Mummy
2007

Dear Baby Raé,

It's so difficult to put into words the amount of love that I have for you. I can never forget finding out that I was pregnant with you and asking God, 'Why?'

Every time I see your beautiful smile and feel your chubby little body in my arms, I am reminded of why God chose me to be your mummy. I know why I was blessed with my wonderful little girl who is so loving, affectionate and cheeky. I want to give you all that I have and encourage and support you in everything you do. You are very special to your daddy, your sister and I and our lives would be incomplete without you.
Keep shining my little 'Raé' of sunshine!

Love you lots,
Mummy
2009

Dear Baby Roman,

You are a very special blessing to me and our family. Ever since I was a little girl I always wanted a son and with you, God answered my prayers.

I have never experienced a love like this before and I know this is because God fulfilled my heart's desires.

I feel so complete and happy. I am so grateful and feel so blessed that I don't want to ever come down from this cloud.

It's so exciting to watch in awe as you do something new each day and I look forward to watching you grow into an amazing young man.

Mummy loves you lots my lil' cubbie.
2014

Published by

Website	www.she-reigns.com
Email	info@she-reigns.co.uk
Instagram	@shereignsltd
Twitter	@shereignsltd
Facebook	She Reigns

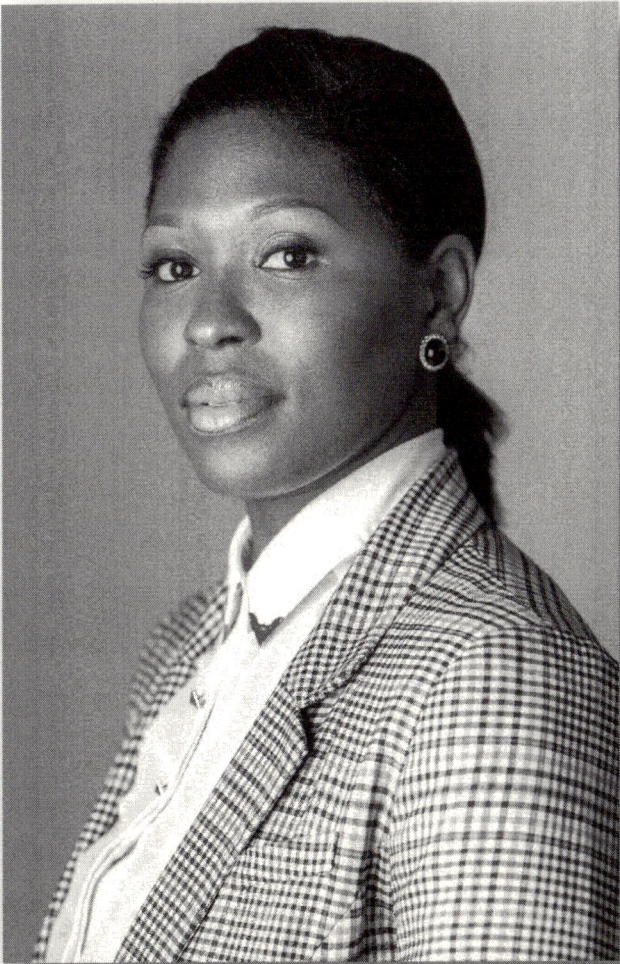